Pescatarian Diet Cookbook

Mouth-Watering Recipes for Your Daily Seafood-Based Meals to Gain Health and Lose weight in The best possible way

Lara Dillard

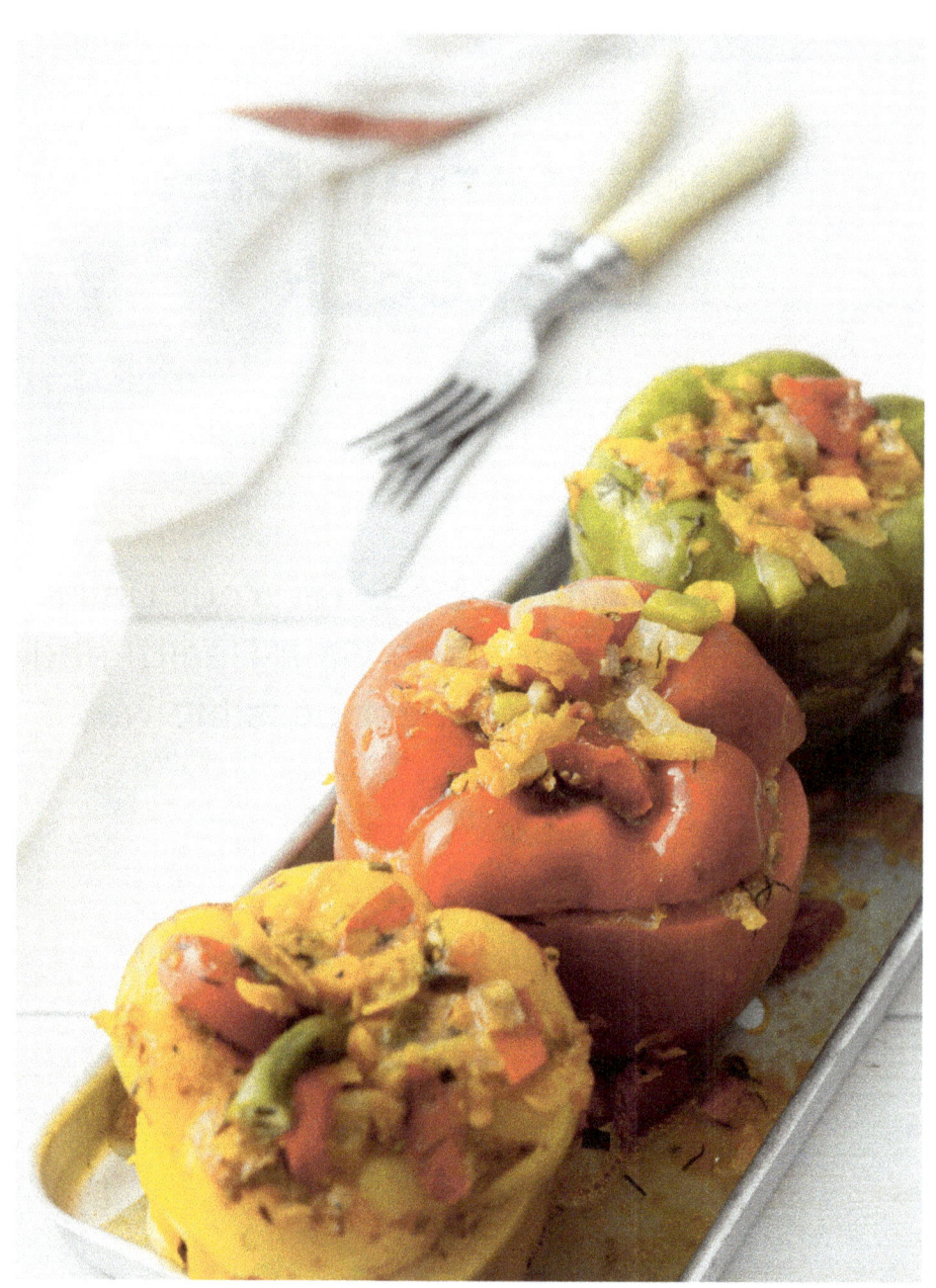

© copyright 2021 – all rights reserved.

the content contained within this book may not be reproduced, duplicated or transmitted without direct written permission from the author or the publisher.

under no circumstances will any blame or legal responsibility be held against the publisher, or author, for any damages, reparation, or monetary loss due to the information contained within this book. either directly or indirectly.

legal notice:

this book is copyright protected. this book is only for personal use. you cannot amend, distribute, sell, use, quote or paraphrase any part, or the content within this book, without the consent of the author or publisher.

disclaimer notice:

please note the information contained within this document is for educational and entertainment purposes only. all effort has been executed to present accurate, up to date, and reliable, complete information. no warranties of any kind are declared or implied. readers acknowledge that the author is not engaging in the rendering of legal, financial, medical or professional advice. the content within this book has been derived from various sources. please consult a licensed professional before attempting any techniques outlined in this book.

by reading this document, the reader agrees that under no circumstances is the author responsible for any losses, direct or indirect, which are incurred as a result of the use of information contained within this document, including, but not limited to, — errors, omissions, or inaccuracies.

Table of Contents

PUMPKIN PASTRY 6
BAKED APPLES 9
BULGARIAN BAKED BEANS 11
RICE STUFFED BELL PEPPERS 13
BEANS STUFFED BELL PEPPERS 15
RED LENTIL FRITTERS 17
SKINNY SOUTHERN BBQ SHRIMP 19
SHRIMP 'N SLAW MARINARA 21
CRANBERRY TUNA SALAD 23
ENGLAND FISH CHOWDER RECIPE 24
FETA OMELETTE 27
TOMATO AND ZUCCHINI DISH 29
SWEET BRUSSELS SPROUTS 31
ROASTED POTATOES 33
FRIED CABBAGE 35
QUINOA SIDE DISH 37
MASHED CAULIFLOWER AND CHIVES 39
CARAMELIZED SWEET POTATOES DISH 42
LEMON GARLIC SALMON 44
CRISPY SHRIMP 46
CREAM OF ZUCCHINI SOUP 48
LOW CARB VEGETABLE SOUP 50
SEAFOOD STEW 52
TUNA AND WHITE BEANS SALAD 54
SHRIMP WITH ONION & PEPPER 56
HAWAIIAN SHRIMP 58
LEMON OLD BAY SHRIMP 60

CHILI HONEY SALMON 62

TENDER & JUICY HONEY GLAZED SALMON 65

EASY HERBED SALMON 68

LEMON BUTTER SALMON.. 70

BONUS AIR FRYER SEAFOOD RECIPES 72

JAPANESE-STYLE FRIED PRAWNS 72

GREAT AIR-FRIED SOFT-SHELL CRAB.. 74

STUNNING AIR-FRIED CLAMS 76

HERBED TROUT AND ASPARAGUS 78

TROUT AND ZUCCHINIS 81

GARLIC BUTTER SHRIMP 82

CAJUN BUTTER SHRIMP... 84

PROSCIUTTO WRAPPED AHI AHI 86

PROSCIUTTO WRAPPED TUNA BITES.. 88

TOMATO PARCHMENT COD 90

ITALIAN STYLE FLOUNDER.. 92

THYME TUNA 94

BUTTERY SHRIMP... 96

MAPLE SALMON 98

HOT PRAWNS 99

TUNA STEAK 101

TROUT WITH BUTTER SAUCE 102

CRAB LEGS IN LEMON BUTTER 104

Pumpkin Pastry

Servings: 8

Ingredients and Quantity

- 14 oz. filo pastry
- 1 cup pumpkin, shredded
- 1 cup walnuts, coarsely chopped
- 1/2 cup sugar
- 6 tbsp. sunflower oil
- 1 tbsp. cinnamon
- 1 tsp. vanilla

Direction

1. Grate the pumpkin and steam it until tender.
2. Cool and add the walnuts, sugar, cinnamon and vanilla.
3. Place a few sheets of pastry in the baking dish.

4.   Sprinkle with oil and spread the filling on top.

5.   Repeat this a few times finishing with a sheet of pastry.

6.   Bake for 20 minutes at 350 degrees F.

7.   Allow the pumpkin pie to cool down and then dust with the powdered sugar. Serve and enjoy!

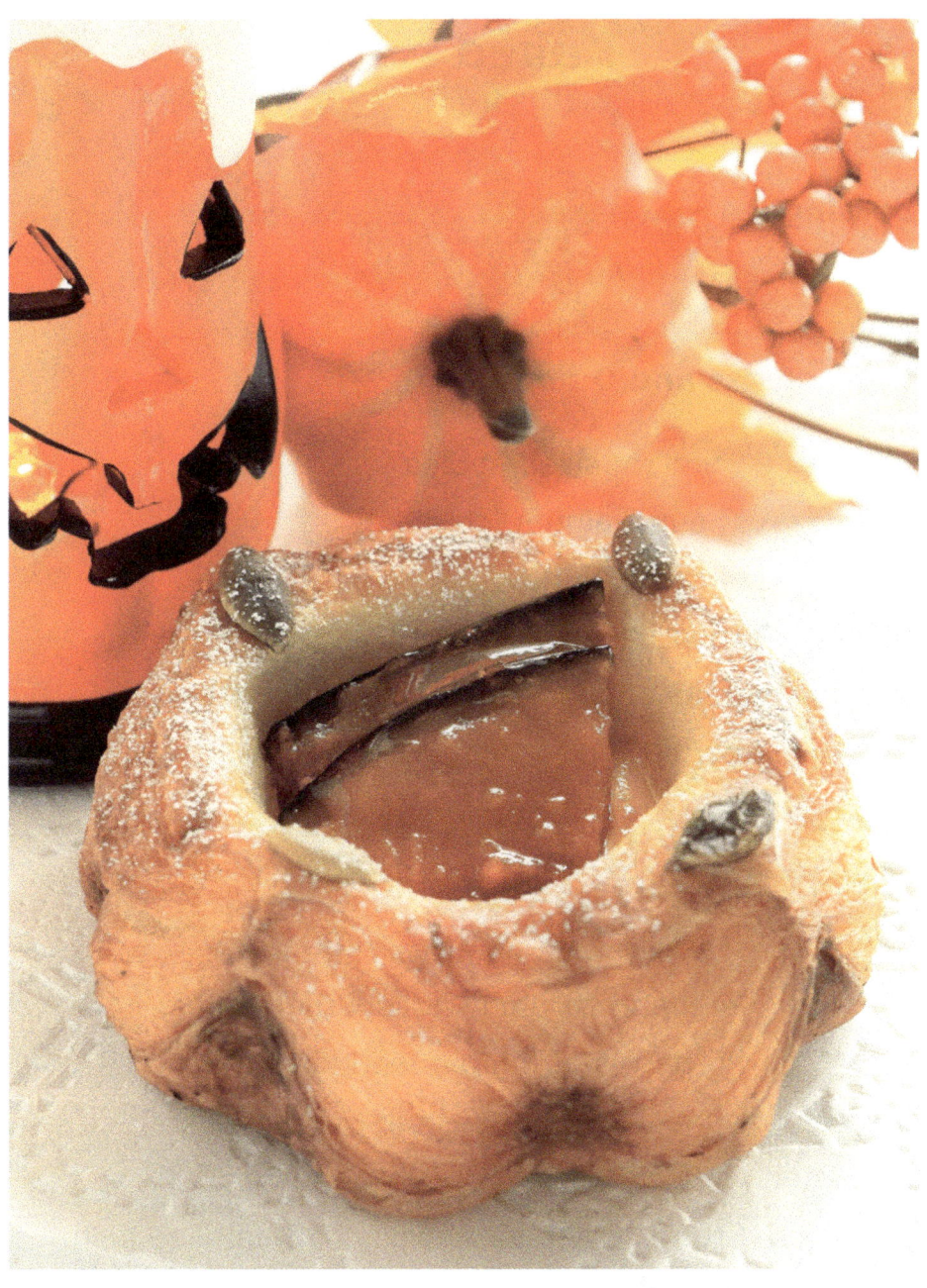

Baked Apples

Servings: 4

Ingredients and Quantity

- 8 medium sized apples
- 1/3 cup walnuts, crushed
- 3/4 cup sugar
- 3 tbsp. raisins, soaked
- Vanilla and cinnamon, to taste
- 2 oz. butter

Direction

1. Peel and carefully hollow the apples.
2. Prepare stuffing by beating butter, 3/4 cup of sugar, crushed walnuts, raisins and cinnamon.
3. Stuff the apples and place in an oiled dish.
4. Pour over 1 to 2 tbsp. of water and bake in a moderate oven.

5. Serve warm with a scoop of vanilla ice cream. Enjoy!

Bulgarian Baked Beans

Servings: 6

Ingredients and Quantity

- 2 cups dried white beans
- 2 medium onions, chopped
- 1 red bell pepper, chopped
- 1 carrot, chopped
- 1/4 cup sunflower oil
- 1 tsp. paprika
- 1 tsp. black pepper
- 1 tbsp. plain flour
- 1/2 bunch fresh parsley and mint
- 1 tsp. salt

Direction

1. Wash the beans and soak in water overnight.
2. In the morning, discard the water, pour enough

cold water to cover the beans.
3. Add one of the onions, peeled and washed but left whole.
4. Cook until the beans are soft but not falling apart.
5. If there is excess water left, drain the beans.
6. Now, chop the other onion and fry it in a frying pan alongside the chopped bell pepper and the carrot.
7. Add paprika, plain flour and the beans.
8. Stir well and pour the mixture in a baking dish along with some parsley, mint and salt.
9. Bake in an oven preheated to 350 degrees F for 20 to 30 minutes.
10. Don't allow the beans to be too dry or too watery.
11. Best served warm. Enjoy!

Rice Stuffed Bell Peppers

Servings: 4

Ingredients and Quantity

- 8 bell peppers, cored and seeded
- 1 1/2 cups rice, washed and drained
- 2 onions, chopped
- 1 tomato, chopped
- Fresh parsley, chopped
- 3 tbsp. olive oil
- 1 tbsp. paprika

Direction

1. Heat the oil and sauté the onions for 2 to 3 minutes.
2. Add the paprika, the washed and rinsed rice, the tomatoes, and then season with salt and pepper.

3. Add 1/2 cup of hot water and cook the rice until the rice is well cooked and the water is absorbed.
4. Stuff each pepper with the mixture using a spoon. Every pepper should be 3/4 full.
5. Arrange the peppers in a deep ovenproof dish and top up with warm water to half fill the dish.
6. Cover and bake for about 20 minutes at 350 degrees F.
7. Uncover and cook for another 15 minutes until the peppers are well cooked.
8. Serve alone or with plain yogurt.

Beans Stuffed Bell Peppers

Servings: 5

Ingredients and Quantity

- 10 dried bell peppers
- 1 cup dried beans
- 1 onion
- 3 garlic cloves
- 2 tbsp. flour
- 1 carrot
- 1 bunch parsley
- 1/2 crushed walnuts
- Some paprika, to taste
- Salt, to taste

Direction

1. Put the dried peppers in warm water and leave them there for 1 hour.
2. Now cook the beans.

3. Chop the carrot and the onion, sauté them and add them to the cooked beans.
4. Add as well the finely chopped parsley and the walnuts.
5. Stir the mixture to make it homogeneous.
6. Drain the peppers, then fill them with the mixture and place in a roasting tin.
7. Cover the pepper's openings with flour to seal them during the baking.
8. Bake them for 30 minutes at 350 degrees F. Serve and enjoy!

Red Lentil Fritters

Servings: 4

Ingredients and Quantity

- 1 cup dry red lentils
- 1/3 cup bulgur
- 3 garlic cloves, crushed
- 5 to 6 spring onions, finely chopped
- 1/2 cup fresh dill, finely cut
- 5 to 6 fresh mint leaves, chopped
- 1 tbsp. tomato paste
- 1 tsp. cumin
- 1 tsp. paprika
- Salt and black pepper, to taste
- 1/2 cup sunflower oil, for frying

Direction

1. Boil lentils in 2 cups of water until the water is almost absorbed.

2. Now add in bulgur and salt. Set aside, covered.
3. When lentil mixture has cooled, add all the other ingredients except the sunflower oil. Stir to combine.
4. Heat the sunflower oil in a frying pan.
5. Drop a few scoops of the lentil mixture and fry them on medium heat, making sure they don't touch.
6. Fry them for 3 to 5 minutes or until golden brown.
7. Serve with vegetable salad. Enjoy!

Skinny Southern BBQ Shrimp

Servings: 4

Ingredients

- 1/4 teaspoon cayenne
- 2 tablespoons Worcestershire sauce
- 1 teaspoon paprika
- 2 teaspoons dried oregano
- 2 teaspoons dried thyme leaves
- Salt and pepper to taste
- 1 pound medium to large peeled shrimp
- 1/3 cup white wine or cooking wine
- 2 tablespoons olive oil
- 2 tablespoons fat-free Caesar or Creamy Italian dressing
- 1 tablespoon minced garlic

Directions

1. Combine oil, Italian dressing, garlic, cayenne, Worcestershire sauce, paprika, oregano, thyme, salt and pepper in large nonstick skillet over medium heat until sauce begins to boil.
2. Add shrimp and cook for 3 to 4 minutes, stirring continuously. Add wine and cook until the shrimp are done, 3 to 5 additional minutes. Serve hot.

Shrimp 'n Slaw Marinara

Servings: 1

Ingredients

- 1/2 cup low-fat marinara sauce
- 4 oz. ready-to-eat shrimp
- One 12-oz. bag (4 cups) broccoli cole slaw
- **For Seasoning:** garlic powder, onion powder, red pepper flakes

Directions

1. Spray a large skillet with nonstick spray to medium-high heat.
2. Add broccoli slaw and 1/2 cup water.
3. Cover and cook until fully softened, about 10 minutes. Uncover and, if needed, cook and stir until water has evaporated, 2 - 3 minutes.

4. Add marinara sauce and shrimp.

5. Cook and stir until hot and well mixed, about 2 minutes. Season to taste!

Cranberry Tuna Salad

Servings: 5

Ingredients

- 1/4 cup red onion, minced
- 1 tbsp. lemon juice
- 1/4 cup dried cranberries
- 1 apple, diced
- Salt and pepper
- 16 oz. can white tuna, packed in water, drained
- 3 tbsp. low fat mayonnaise
- 3 tbsp. light sour cream
- 1/2 cup celery, chopped

Directions

1. Combine all the ingredients. Season with salt and pepper
2. Serve right away!

3. Refrigerate if not eating right away.

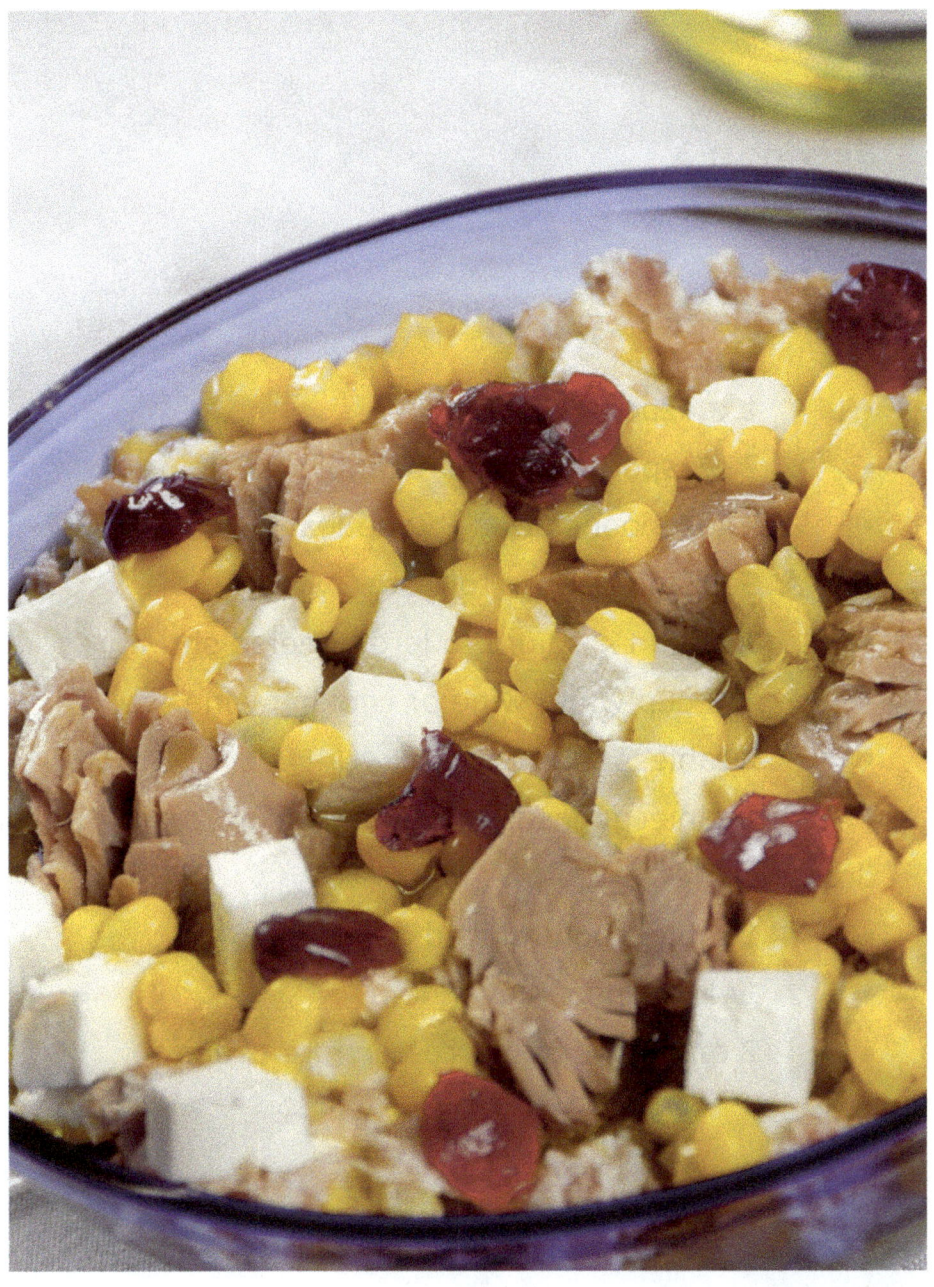

England Fish Chowder Recipe

Servings: 3

Ingredients

- 1 teaspoon paprika
- 2 teaspoons dried oregano
- 2 teaspoons dried thyme leaves
- Salt and pepper to taste
- 1 pound medium to large peeled shrimp
- 1/3 cup white wine or cooking wine
- 2 tablespoons olive oil
- 2 tablespoons fat-free Caesar or Creamy Italian dressing
- 1 tablespoon minced garlic
- 1/4 teaspoon cayenne
- 2 tablespoons Worcestershire sauce

Directions

1. Combine oil, Italian dressing, garlic, cayenne, Worcestershire sauce, paprika, oregano, thyme, salt and pepper in large nonstick skillet over medium heat until sauce begins to boil.
2. Add shrimp and cook for 3 to 4 minutes, stirring continuously.
3. Add wine and cook until the shrimp are done, 3 to 5 additional minutes. Serve hot.

Feta Omelette

Servings: 5

Ingredients and Quantity

- 1 small onion, finely cut
- 1 green bell pepper, chopped
- 1 red pepper, chopped
- 4 tomatoes, cubed
- 2 garlic cloves, crushed
- 8 eggs
- 10 oz. feta cheese, crumbled
- 4 tbsp. olive oil
- 1/2 bunch parsley
- Black pepper and salt, to taste

Direction

1. In a large pan, sauté onion over medium heat, till transparent.
2. Reduce the heat and add bell peppers and garlic.
3. Continue cooking until soft.

4. Add the tomatoes and continue simmering until the mixture is almost dry.
5. Add the cheese and all the eggs.
6. Stir and cook well until well mixed and not too watery.
7. Season with black pepper and remove from heat.
8. Sprinkle with parsley. Serve and enjoy!

Tomato and Zucchini Dish

Servings: 3

Total Time: 20 Minutes

Calories: 70

Fat: 1 g

Protein: 2 g

Carbs: 6 g

Fiber: 2.8 g

Ingredients and Quantity

- Salt and black pepper, to taste
- 2 garlic cloves, minced
- 6 zucchinis, chopped
- A drizzle olive oil
- 1 tbsp. vegetable oil
- 1 pound colored cherry tomatoes

- 2 yellow onion, chopped
- 1 cup tomato puree
- 1 bunch basil, finely chopped
-

Direction

1. Heat up a pan with the vegetable oil over medium high heat and add onions. Stir and sauté those for 5 minutes.
2. Transfer this to your instant pot, add zucchini, tomatoes, salt, pepper, and tomato puree.
3. Cover and cook on High for 5 minutes.
4. Release pressure naturally, add garlic and basil, more salt and pepper if needed and a drizzle of olive oil.
5. Toss to coat, divide amongst plates and serve. Enjoy!

Sweet Brussels Sprouts

Servings: 8

Total Time: 15 Minutes

Calories: 193

Fat: 4 g

Protein: 10 g

Carbs: 8 g

Fiber: 1 g

Ingredients and Quantity

- 1 tsp. oregano zest, grated
- 1/4 cup orange juice
- 2 pounds Brussels sprouts, trimmed
- 1 tbsp. olive oil
- 2 tbsp. stevia
- A pinch salt and black pepper

Direction

1. Set your instant pot on Sauté mode. Add oil and heat it up.
2. Add the sprouts, stir and cook on medium high for 1 minute.
3. Add orange zest, orange juice, stevia, salt and pepper.
4. Stir, cover and cook on High for 4 minutes.
5. Divide between plates. Serve and enjoy right away!

Roasted Potatoes

Servings: 4

Total Time: 25 Minutes

Calories: 190

Fat: 6 g

Protein: 9 g

Carbs: 10 g

Fiber: 8 g

Ingredients and Quantity

- 1/2 tsp. onion powder
- 1/4 tsp. sweet paprika
- 1 1/2 pounds potatoes, cut into wedges
- 1/4 cup avocado oil
- A pinch salt and black pepper
- 1 cup veggie stock
- 1 tsp. garlic powder

Direction

1. Add the oil to your instant pot. Set it to Sauté mode and heat the oil up.
2. Add potatoes and cook them for 8 minutes.
3. Add salt, pepper, onion powder, garlic powder, paprika and stock.
4. Toss a bit, cover pot and cook on High for 7 minutes.
5. Divide potatoes amongst plates. Serve and enjoy!

Fried Cabbage

Servings: 4

Total Time: 16 Minutes

Calories: 200

Fat: 4 g

Protein: 5 g

Carbs: 8 g

Fiber: 1 g

Ingredients and Quantity

- 2 tsp. balsamic vinegar
- 3 garlic cloves, minced
- 1 tbsp. olive oil
- 1 cabbage head, sliced
- 1 yellow onion, chopped
- 2 tsp. stevia

- A pinch salt and black pepper
- 2 tsp. mustard

Direction

1. Set your instant pot on Sauté mode. Add oil and heat it up.
2. Add onion and garlic. Stir and sauté for 2 minutes.
3. Add cabbage, stevia, vinegar, mustard, salt and pepper.
4. Stir, cover and cook on High for 4 minutes.
5. Stir cabbage one more time. Divide amongst plates. Serve and enjoy!

Quinoa Side Dish

Servings: 4

Total Time: 12 Minutes

Calories: 182

Fat: 4 g

Protein: 10 g

Carbs: 8 g

Fiber: 2 g

Ingredients and Quantity

- Juice of 1 lemon
- A pinch salt and black pepper
- 2 cups quinoa
- 3 cups water
- A handful parsley, cilantro and basil, chopped

Direction

1. In your instant pot, mix quinoa with water, lemon, salt, pepper and mixed herbs.
2. Stir, cover and cook on High for 2 minutes.
3. Leave quinoa aside for 10 minutes. Fluff with a fork.
4. Divide amongst plates. Serve and enjoy!

Mashed Cauliflower and Chives

Servings: 4

Total Time: 16 Minutes

Calories: 200

Fat: 4 g

Protein: 10 g

Carbs: 7 g

Fiber: 4 g

Ingredients and Quantity

- 2 tsp. olive oil
- A pinch salt and black pepper
- 1/2 tsp. turmeric powder
- 1 1/2 cups water
- 1/2 cups water
- 1 cauliflower head, florets separated
- 3 chives, chopped

Direction

1. Put the water in your instant pot. Add steamer basket and then put the cauliflower inside.
2. Cover and cook on High for 6 minutes.
3. Transfer cauliflower to a bowl. Mash with a potato masher and transfer to your food processor.
4. Add salt, pepper, chives, turmeric and oil. Blend well.
5. Divide amongst serving plates. Serve and enjoy!

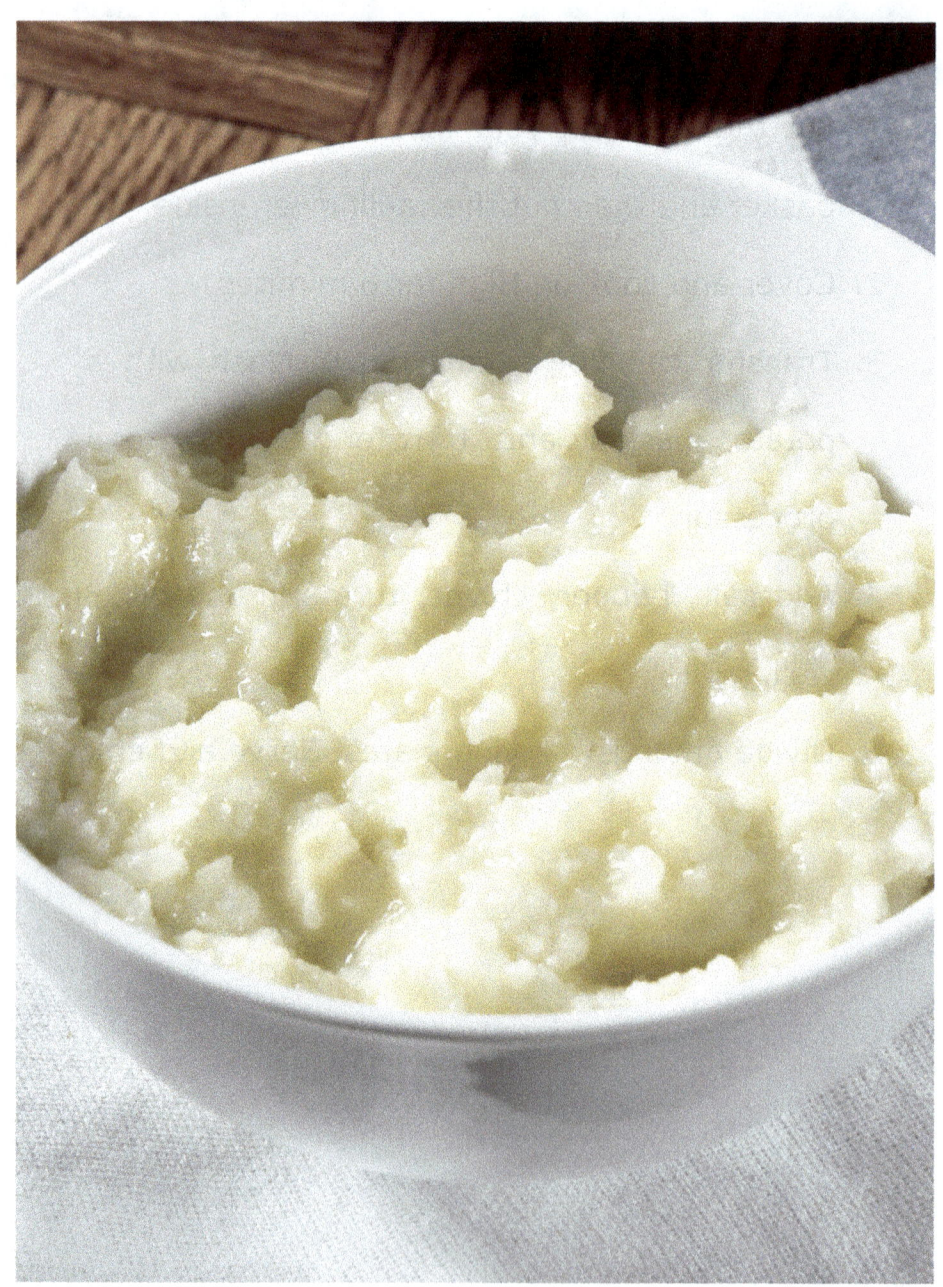

Caramelized Sweet Potatoes Dish

Servings: 4

Total Time: 30 Minutes

Calories: 182

Fat: 5 g

Protein: 9 g

Carbs: 9 g

Fiber: 5 g

Ingredients and Quantity

- 1 cup water
- A pinch salt and black pepper
- 2 tbsp. coconut oil
- 2 sweet potatoes, scrubbed
- pinch chili powder

Direction

1. Add the water to your instant pot. Add steamer basket and then put the sweet potatoes.
2. Cover and cook on High for 15 minutes.
3. Transfer potatoes to a cutting board and slice them.
4. Clean your instant pot, set it on Sauté mode. Add oil, heat it up.
5. Add sweet potato slices, season with salt, pepper and chili powder and brown them for 2 minutes on each side.
6. Divide between plates and serve. Enjoy!

Lemon Garlic Salmon

Servings: 2

Total Time: 10 Minutes

Calories: 538

Fat: 28.8 g

Protein: 58.5 g

Carbs: 3.3 g

Fiber: 0.9 g

Ingredients and Quantity

- 1 1/2 pounds frozen salmon fillets
- 1/4 cup lemon juice
- 3/4 cup fish stock or water
- 1 lemon, thinly sliced
- 1 tbsp. coconut oil
- 2 tbsp. mixed herbs

- 1 tsp. garlic powder
- 1 tsp. salt
- 1 tsp. black pepper
-

Direction

1. Add the lemon juice, fish stock, and mixed herbs to your Instant Pot.
2. Place a steamer rack in Instant Pot.
3. Drizzle the salmon fillets with coconut oil and season with garlic powder, salt, and black pepper.
4. Place the salmon on the steamer rack and place lemon slices on top.
5. Lock the lid and cook at high pressure for 7 minutes.
6. When the cooking is done, quick release the pressure and remove the lid. Serve and enjoy!

Crispy Shrimp

Servings: 4

Total Time: 30 Minutes

Calories: 229

Fat: 4.9 g

Protein: 30.7 g

Carbs: 13.8 g

Ingredients and Quantity

- 1 lb. shrimp, peeled and deveined
- 4 tbsp. apple sauce
- 1/2 cup bread crumbs
- 1/2 cup onion, diced
- 1 tsp. ginger1 tsp. garlic powder
- Salt and pepper, to taste

Direction

1. In one bowl, beat the two eggs.
2. In another bowl, put the rest of the ingredients.
3. Dip the shrimp first in the apple sauce and then in the spice mixture.
4. Place in the Ninja Foodi basket.
5. Seal the crisping lid.
6. Choose air crisp function.
7. Cook at 350 degrees for 10 minutes.
8. You can serve with chili sauce. Enjoy!

Cream of Zucchini Soup

Servings: 4

Total Time: 5 Hours 10 Minutes

Calories: 79

Fat: 10 g

Protein: 5 g

Carbs: 4.3 g

Ingredients and Quantity

- 1 tbsp. coconut cream
- 1/4 tbsp. pepper
- 1 tbsp. almond butter
- 1/2 cup chopped yellow onion
- 2 cups vegetable broth
- 4 cups chopped with peel green zucchini squash

Direction

1. Mix all the ingredients in your crock pot just leaving out the coconut cream.
2. Cook for about 5 hours on low or until zucchini is tender-soft.
3. Puree the soup in a blender.
4. Stir in the coconut cream then serve. Enjoy!

Low Carb Vegetable Soup

Servings: 6

Total Time: 8 Hours 10 Minutes

Calories: 125.2

Fat: 3.9 g

Protein: 11.9 g

Carbs: 11.6 g

Ingredients and Quantity

- 8 oz. fresh mushrooms, sliced
- 2 cans (14 oz.) vegetable broth
- 1 can diced tomatoes
- 1 green pepper, chopped
- 1 yellow onion, chopped
- 1 zucchini, thinly sliced
- 4 oz. turkey, sliced
- Vegan cheese, for topping

- 1 tsp. stevia
- 1 1/2 tbsp. basil leaves
- 1/2 tsp. salt

Direction

1. Put the broth, veggies, tomatoes, stevia, salt and basil in a slow cooker and mix thoroughly.
2. Top with the turkey slices then cook on low for 8 hours or high for 4 hours.
3. Pour into bowls and top with the cheese. Serve and enjoy!

Seafood Stew

Servings: 6

Total Time: 8 Hours 10 Minutes

Calories: 117.4

Fat: 5.8 g

Protein: 25.2 g

Carbs: 4.7 g

Ingredients and Quantity

- 2 tbsp. fresh parsley, chopped
- 1/2 tsp. salt
- 1 tsp. dried basil leaves
- 1/4 tsp. red pepper sauce
- 2 tbsp. olive oil
- 1 cup baby carrots, sliced
- 3 cups sliced quartered Roma tomatoes
- 1 tsp. Splenda

- 1/2 cup green bell pepper, chopped
- 1 cup water
- 1/2 tsp. fennel seed
- 1/2 lb. peeled and deveined shrimp
- 1 lb. cod cut into 1 inch slices
- 2 garlic cloves, finely chopped

Direction

1. Mix garlic and oil in a crockpot. Add tomatoes, carrots, fennel seed, bell pepper, clam juice and water then stir.
2. Cover and cook for 8 to 9 hours on low heat or until the vegetables are tender.
3. Around 20 minutes before serving, stir in the shrimp, cod, basil, splenda, pepper sauce and salt.
4. Cover and cook on high until the fish flakes with a fork.
5. Add in the parsley and stir. Serve and enjoy!

Tuna and White Beans Salad

Servings: 6

Total Time: 9 Hours 15 Minutes

Calories: 468

Fat: 15.5 g

Protein: 35.8 g

Carbs: 48.4 g

Ingredients and Quantity

- 4 tbsp. extra virgin olive oil
- 1 garlic clove, crushed and minced
- 1 lb. white beans, soaked overnight, rinsed and drained
- 6 cups water
- 14 oz. canned white tuna in water, drained and shredded
- 2 cups tomatoes, chopped

- 2 tsp. dried basil
- Salt and pepper, to taste
- 1 bunch Romaine lettuce, chopped

Direction

1. Add the olive oil to a skillet. Sauté the garlic for 1 minute.
2. Remove the garlic from the pan.
3. Cook the beans in the slow cooker on low for 3 hours.
4. Add the garlic-flavored olive oil.
5. Pour the water into the pot.
6. Cover and set it on high. Cook for 1 hour.
7. Reduce the temperature to low.
8. Cook for another 5 hours.
9. Add the tuna, tomatoes and basil. Mix well.
10. Arrange the lettuce in salad bowls.
11. Top with the tuna and beans mixture. Serve and enjoy!

Shrimp with Onion & Pepper

Preparation Time: 10 minutes

Cooking Time: 15 minutes

Serve: 4

Nutritional Value (Amount per Serving):

- Calories 183
- Fat 5.6 g
- Carbohydrates 5.9 g
- Sugar 2.2 g

- Protein 26.4 g
- Cholesterol 239 mg

Ingredients:

- 1 lb shrimp, peeled & deveined
- 1/8 tsp cayenne

- 1/2 tsp garlic powder
- 1 tsp chili powder
- 1 tbsp olive oil
- 1/2 onion, cut into chunks
- 1 bell pepper, cut into chunks
- Pepper
- Salt

Directions:

1. Add shrimp and remaining ingredients into the bowl and toss well.
2. Add shrimp mixture into the air fryer basket and cook at 330 F for 15 minutes. Stir halfway through.
3. Serve and enjoy.

Hawaiian Shrimp

Preparation Time: 10 minutes

Cooking Time: 8 minutes

Serve: 4

Nutritional Value (Amount per Serving):

- Calories 257
- Fat 13.5 g
- Carbohydrates 6.5 g
- Sugar 0.1 g
- Protein 26.2 g
- Cholesterol 269 mg

Ingredients:

- 1 lb shrimp
- 1 1/2 tsp paprika
- 2 tbsp cornstarch

- 1 tbsp garlic, minced
- 1/4 cup butter
- Pepper
- Salt

Directions:

1. Add shrimp, cornstarch, paprika, pepper, and salt into the bowl and toss until well coated.
2. Spray air fryer basket with cooking spray.
3. Add shrimp into the air fryer basket and cook at 350 F for 8 minutes.
4. Melt butter in a pan over medium heat, once butter is melted then add garlic and sauté for 30 seconds.
5. Pour garlic butter mixture over shrimp and serve.

Lemon Old Bay Shrimp

Preparation Time: 10 minutes

Cooking Time: 10 minutes

Serve: 4

Nutritional Value (Amount per Serving):

- Calories 148
- Fat 3.4 g
- Carbohydrates 1.9 g
- Sugar 0 g
- Protein 25.9 g
- Cholesterol 243 mg

Ingredients:

- 1 lb shrimp, peeled & deveined
- 1 tbsp old bay seasoning
- 1/2 tsp garlic, minced

- 1/2 tsp lemon juice
- 1/2 tbsp butter, melted
- Pepper
- Salt

Directions:

1. Add shrimp and remaining ingredients into the bowl and toss well.
2. Add shrimp mixture into the air fryer basket and cook at 390 F for 8-10 minutes. Stir halfway through.
3. Serve and enjoy.

Chili Honey Salmon

Preparation Time: 10 minutes

Cooking Time: 12 minutes

Serve: 2

Nutritional Value (Amount per Serving):

- Calories 336
- Fat 11.2 g
- Carbohydrates 26.8 g
- Sugar 26 g
- Protein 34.8 g
- Cholesterol 78 mg

Ingredients:

- 2 salmon fillets
- 3 tbsp honey
- 1/2 tbsp chili flakes

- 1/2 tsp chili powder
- 1/2 tsp turmeric
- 1 tsp ground coriander
- 1/8 tsp pepper
- 1/8 tsp salt

Directions:

1. Add honey to microwave-safe bowl and heat for 10 seconds.
2. Add chili flakes, chili powder, turmeric, coriander, pepper, and salt into the honey and mix well.
3. Brush salmon fillets with honey mixture.
4. Place salmon fillets into the air fryer basket and cook at 400 F for 12 minutes.
5. Serve and enjoy.

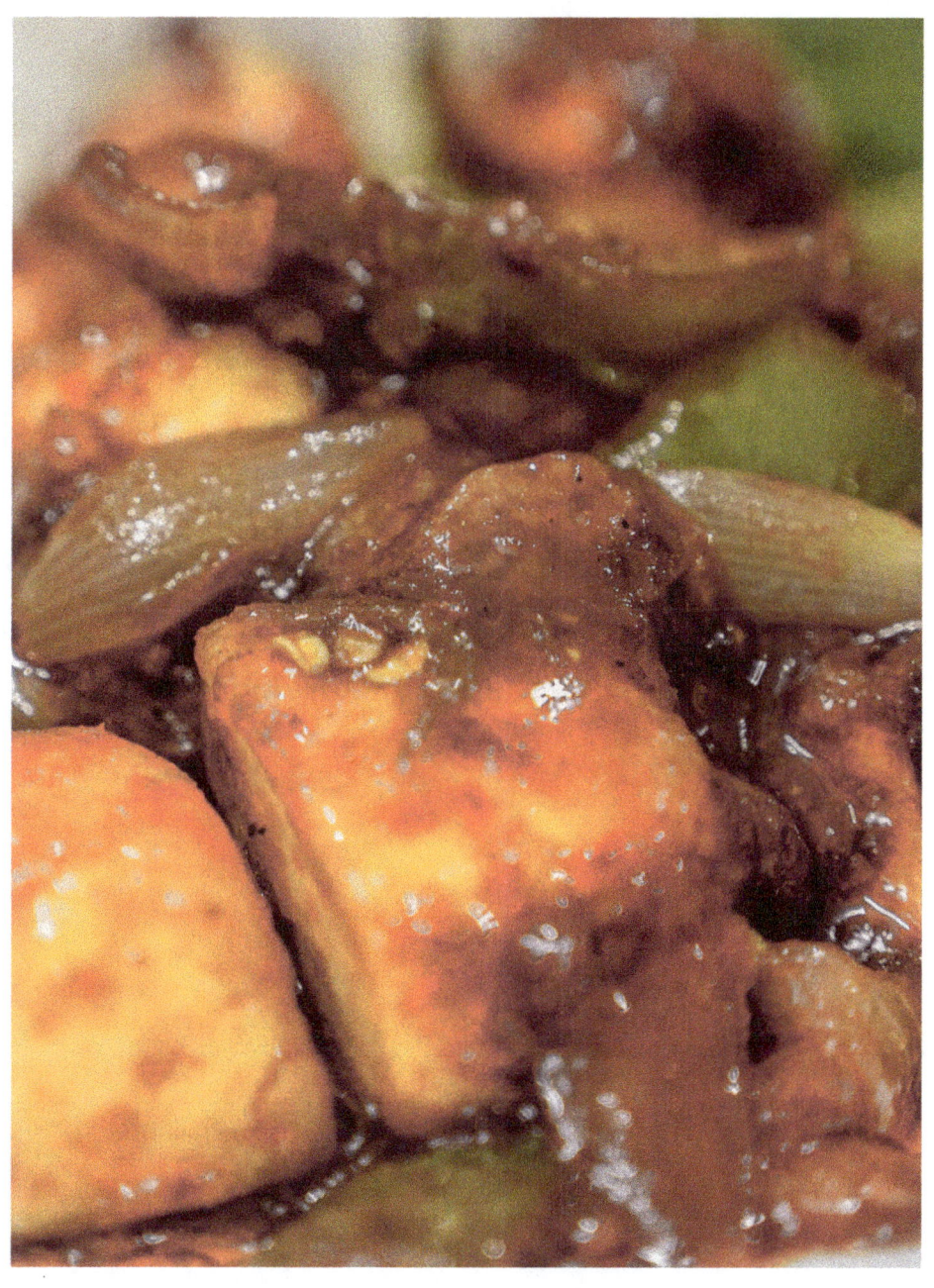

Tender & Juicy Honey Glazed Salmon

Preparation Time: 10 minutes

Cooking Time: 10 minutes

Serve: 4

Nutritional Value (Amount per Serving):

- Calories 271
- Fat 13.1 g
- Carbohydrates 4.5 g
- Sugar 4.3 g
- Protein 34.7 g
- Cholesterol 78 mg

Ingredients:

- 4 salmon fillets

- 1 tbsp honey
- 1/2 tsp red chili flakes, crushed
- 1 tsp sesame seeds, toasted
- 1 1/2 tsp olive oil
- 1 tbsp coconut aminos
- Pepper
- Salt

Direction

1. Place salmon fillets into the bowl. In a small bowl, mix coconut aminos, oil, pepper, and salt and pour over fish fillets. Mix well.
2. Cover bowl and place in the refrigerator for 20 minutes.
3. Preheat the air fryer to 400 F.
4. Place marinated salmon fillets into the air fryer basket and cook for 8 minutes.

5. Brush fish fillets with honey and sprinkle with chili flakes and sesame seeds and cook for 2 minutes more.

6. Serve and enjoy.

Easy Herbed Salmon

Preparation Time: 10 minutes

Cooking Time: 5 minutes

Serve: 2

Nutritional Value (Amount per Serving):

- Calories 407
- Fat 30.8 g
- Carbohydrates 0.2 g
- Sugar 0 g
- Protein 34.6 g
- Cholesterol 94 mg

Ingredients:

- 2 salmon fillets
- 1 tbsp butter
- 2 tbsp olive oil

- 1/4 tsp paprika
- 1 tsp herb de Provence
- Pepper
- Salt

Directions:

1. Brush salmon fillets with oil and sprinkle with paprika, herb de Provence, pepper, and salt.
2. Place salmon fillets into the air fryer basket and cook at 390 F for 5 minutes.
3. Melt butter in a pan and pour over cooked salmon fillets.
4. Serve and enjoy.

Lemon Butter Salmon

Preparation Time: 10 minutes

Cooking Time: 12 minutes

Serve: 2

Nutritional Value (Amount per Serving):

- Calories 344
- Fat 22.6 g
- Carbohydrates 1.1 g
- Sugar 0.3 g
- Protein 35 g
- Cholesterol 109 mg

Ingredients:

- 2 salmon fillets
- 1/2 tsp soy sauce
- 3/4 tsp dill, chopped

- 1 tsp garlic, minced
- 1 1/2 tbsp fresh lemon juice
- 2 tbsp butter, melted
- Pepper
- Salt

Directions:

1. Preheat the air fryer to 400 F.
2. In a small bowl, mix butter, lemon juice, garlic, dill, soy sauce, pepper, and salt.
3. Brush salmon fillets with butter mixture and place into the air fryer basket and cook for 10-12 minutes.
4. Pour the remaining butter mixture over cooked salmon fillets and serve.

Bonus Air Fryer Seafood Recipes

Japanese-Style Fried Prawns

Servings: 2

- 1pound of peeled and deveined prawns
- 1cup of rice flour
- 1cup of panko breadcrumbs
- 2 eggs
- 1teaspoon of ground ginger
- 1 tablespoon of paprika
- 1teaspoon of salt
- **1**teaspoon of black pepper
- 1 teaspoon of garlic powder

Directions:

1. Preheat your air fryer to 380 degrees fahrenheit.
2. Using a bowl, add the prawns, salt, black pepper, garlic powder, ground ginger and toss until it is properly mixed.
3. Then using another bowl, add the rice flour

paprika and mix it well. Pick a second bowl, add the eggs and beat it properly. Then using a third bowl, add the panko breadcrumbs.

4. Dredge the seasoned prawns into the flour, dip it into the egg wash, and then cover it with the panko breadcrumbs.

5. Grease your air fryer basket with a nonstick Cooking spray and add the prawns.

6. Cook it for 8 minutes or until it has a golden-brown color and repeat if necessary.

7. Serve and enjoy!

Great Air-Fried Soft-Shell Crab

Servings: 2

- 2soft-shell crabs 1 cup of flour
- 2beaten eggs
- 1cup of panko breadcrumbs
- 1 teaspoon of onion powder
- 1 teaspoon of garlic powder
- 1 teaspoon of salt
- 1teaspoon of black pepper

Directions:

1. Preheat your air fryer to 360 degrees fahrenheit.
2. Use a bowl, add the flour, pick a second bowl, and add the eggs and mix properly. Then using a third bowl, mix the panko breadcrumbs and the seasonings properly.
3. Grease your air fryer basket with a nonstick Cooking spray and add the crabs inside.
4. Cook it inside your air fryer for 8 minutes or until it has a goldenbrown color.
5. After that, carefully remove it from your air fryer and

allow it to cool off.

6. Serve and enjoy!

Stunning Air-Fried Clams

Servings: 2

- 1(10-ounce) can of whole baby clams, drained and shucked
- 2 beaten eggs
- 1cup of flour
- 1cup of panko breadcrumbs
- 1 teaspoon of salt
- 1teaspoon of black pepper
- 1 teaspoon of garlic powder
- 1teaspoon of onion powder
- 1 teaspoon of cayenne pepper
- 1tablespoon of dried oregano

Directions:

Preheat your air fryer to 390 degrees fahrenheit.

Use a bowl, add the flour, pick a second bowl, and add the eggs and mix properly. Using a third bowl, add and mix the panko breadcrumbs, seasonings, and the herbs properly.

Dredge the clams in the flour, immerse it into the egg wash and

then cover it with the breadcrumb mixture.

Place the clams inside your air fryer and cook it for 2 minutes or until it has a golden-brown color, while being cautious of overCooking .

After that, carefully remove it from your air fryer and allow it to cool.

Serve and enjoy!

Herbed Trout And Asparagus

Servings: 4

- 4 trout fillets; boneless and skinless
- 1 bunch asparagus; trimmed
- ¼ cup mixed chives and tarragon
- 2 tbsp. Ghee; melted
- tbsp. Olive oil
- 1 tbsp. Lemon juice
- A pinch of salt and black pepper

Directions:

1. Mix the asparagus with half of the oil, salt and pepper, put it in your air fryer's basket, cook at 380°f for 6 minutes and divide between plates
2. Take a bowl and mix the trout with salt, pepper, lemon juice, the rest of the oil and the herbs and toss,
3. Put the fillets in your air fryer's basket and cook at 380°f for 7 minutes on each side

4.Divide the fish next to the asparagus, drizzle the melted ghee all over and serve

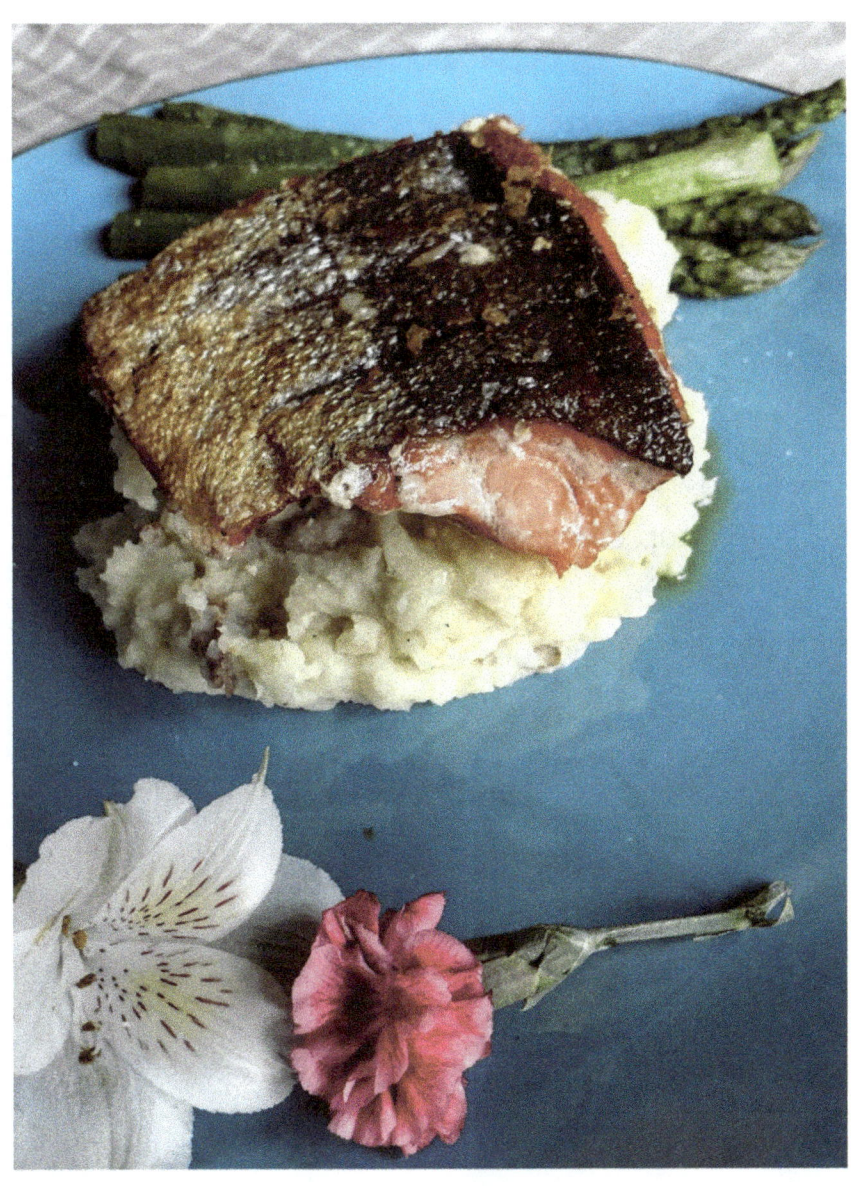

Trout And Zucchinis

Servings: 4

- 3zucchinis, cut in medium chunks
- 4 trout fillets; boneless
- ¼ cup tomato sauce
- 1garlic clove; minced
- ½ cup cilantro; chopped.
- 1 tbsp. Lemon juice
- 2tbsp. Olive oil
- Salt and black pepper to taste.

Directions:

1. In a pan that fits your air fryer, mix the fish with the other , toss, introduce in the fryer and cook at 380°f for 15 minutes.
2. Divide everything between plates and serve right away

Garlic Butter Shrimp

Servings: 4

- 1-pound shrimp, cleaned completely
- 5 tbsp butter, melted
- ½ tsp ground black pepper
- ½ tsp salt
- ½ cup vegetable stock
- 2 tbsp lemon juice
- ¼ cup minced garlic
- 2 tbsp parsley

Directions:

Preheat your air fryer to 350 degrees f and line the air fryer tray or baking pan with foil.

Place the shrimp, butter, pepper, salt, vegetable stock, and garlic in a large bowl and toss together well. Pour the mix onto the prepared tray or pan.

Bake for 12 minutes, stirring occasionally to flip the shrimp.

Divide on to plates and garnish with the lemon juice and garlic. Enjoy hot!

Cajun Butter Shrimp

Servings: 4

- 1-pound shrimp, cleaned completely
- 5 tbsp butter, melted
- ½ tsp ground black pepper
- ½ tsp salt
- tsp cajun seasoning
- ½ cup vegetable stock
- 2 tbsp lemon juice
- tbsp parsley

Directions:

1. Preheat your air fryer to 350 degrees f and line the air fryer tray or baking pan with foil.
2. Place the shrimp, butter, pepper, salt, cajun seasoning and vegetable stock in a large bowl and toss together well. Pour the mix onto the prepared tray or pan.
3. Bake for 12 minutes, stirring occasionally to flip the shrimp.

4.Divide on to plates and garnish with the lemon juice and garlic. Enjoy hot!

Prosciutto Wrapped Ahi Ahi

Servings: 2

- 1-pound cod ahi ahi
- ¼ tsp salt
- ¼ tsp ground black pepper
- 2oz prosciutto de parma, very thinly sliced
- 2 tbsp olive oil
- **1**tsp minced garlic
- 4 cups baby spinach
- 2 tsp lemon juice

Directions:

1. Preheat your air fryer to 325 degrees f and line your air fryer tray
2. with foil.
3. Dry the cod fillets by patting with a paper towel the sprinkle with salt and pepper.
4. Wrap the filets in the prosciutto, enclosing

them as fully as possible.

5. Place the wrapped filets on the prepared tray.

6. Place the tray in the air fryer and bake for 10 minutes.

7. Toss the spinach with the olive oil, garlic and lemon juice andremove the tray from the air fryer and place the spinach mix on the tray as well, around the wrapped cod.

8. Place in the air fryer and bake for another 10 minutes. The spinach should be nicely wilted and the fish 145 degrees f internally.

9. Serve hot!

Prosciutto Wrapped Tuna Bites

Servings: 2

- 1-pound tuna cut into 1" pieces
- ¼ tsp salt
- ¼ tsp ground black pepper
- 2oz prosciutto de parma, very thinly sliced
- 2 tbsp olive oil
- tsp minced garlic
- 4 cups baby spinach
- 2 tsp lemon juice

Directions:

1. Preheat your air fryer to 325 degrees f and line your air fryer tray with foil.
2. Dry the tuna bites by patting with a paper towel the sprinkle with salt and pepper.
3. Wrap the bites in the prosciutto, enclosing them as fully as possible.
4. Place the wrapped bites on the prepared tray.

5. Toss the spinach with the olive oil, garlic and lemon juice and place on the tray as well, around the wrapped tuna.

6. Place in the air fryer and bake for 12 minutes. The spinach should be nicely wilted and the fish 145 degrees f internally.

7. Serve hot!

Tomato Parchment Cod

Servings: 5

- 1¾ pound cod fillets
- ¼ tsp salt
- 1tsp smoked paprika
- 1tsp ground dried ginger
- ¼ cup pitted olives
- ¼ cup sundried tomatoes
- ¼ cup capers
- 1tbsp fresh chopped dill
- 1/3 cup keto marinara

Directions:

1. Preheat your air fryer to 400 degrees f and line your air fryer tray
2. with a long piece of parchment paper.
3. Place the cod filets on the parchment and sprinkle with the salt, paprika, ginger, and rub the fish's

spices.

4.Top the fish with the remaining and then wrap the parchment paper around the fish filets, enclosing them completely.

5.Place the tray in the a. fryer and bake for 15 minutes.

6.Remove from the air fryer, unwrap the parchment and serve while hot!

Italian Style Flounder

Servings: 5

- 1¾ pound salmon fillets
- ¼ tsp salt
- tsp italian seasoning
- 1 cup baby spinach
- ¼ cup sundried tomatoes
- 1 tbsp fresh chopped dill
- 1/3 cup keto pesto sauce

Directions:

1. Preheat your air fryer to 400 degrees f and line your air fryer tray with a long piece of parchment paper.
2. Place the flounder filets on the parchment and sprinkle with the salt and italian seasoning and rub the fish's spices.
3. Top the fish with the remaining and then wrap the parchment paper around the fish filets, enclosing them

completely.

4.Place the tray in the air fryer and bake for 20 minutes.

Remove from the air fryer, unwrap the parchment and serve while hot!

Thyme Tuna

Servings: 4

- ½ cup cilantro, chopped
- ⅓ cup olive oil
- 1 small red onion, chopped
- 3 tablespoons balsamic vinegar
- 2 tablespoons parsley, chopped
- 2 tablespoons basil, chopped
- 1 jalapeno pepper, chopped
- 4 sushi tuna steaks
- Salt and black pepper to taste
- 1 teaspoon red pepper flakes
- teaspoon thyme, chopped
- garlic cloves, minced

Directions:

1. Place all except the fish into a bowl and stir well.
2. Add the fish and toss, coating it well.
3. Transfer everything to your air fryer and cook at

360 degrees f for 4 minutes on each side.

4.Divide the fish between plates and serve.

Buttery Shrimp

Servings: 2

- 1tablespoon butter, melted
- A drizzle of olive oil
- 1-pound shrimp, peeled and deveined
- ¼ cup heavy cream
- 8ounces mushrooms, roughly sliced
- A pinch of red pepper flakes
- Salt and black pepper to taste
- 2 garlic cloves, minced
- ½ cup beef stock
- tablespoon parsley, chopped
- 1 tablespoon chives, chopped

Directions:

1. Season the shrimp with salt and pepper and grease with the oil.
2. Place the shrimp in your air fryer, cook at 360 degrees f for 7 minutes, and divide between plates.
3. Heat a pan with the butter over medium heat, add the

mushrooms, stir, and cook for 3-4 minutes.

4.Add all remaining ; stir and then cook for a few minutes more.

5.Drizzle the butter / garlic mixture over the shrimp and serve.

Maple Salmon

Servings: 2

- 2 salmon fillets, boneless
- Salt and black pepper to taste
- 2 tablespoons mustard
- 1 tablespoon olive oil
- 1 tablespoon maple syrup

Directions:

1. In a bowl, mix the mustard with the oil and the maple syrup; whisk well and brush the salmon with this mix.
2. Place the salmon in your air fryer and cook it at 370 degrees f for 5
3. minutes on each side.
4. Serve immediately with a side salad.

Hot Prawns

Servings: 2

- 6prawns
- ½ teaspoon chili powder
- 1 teaspoon chili flakes
- ¼ teaspoon black pepper
- ¼ teaspoon salt

Directions:

1. preheat the air fryer to 350f.

2. in a bowl, add prawns and spices and mix well.

3. spray air fryer basket with Cooking spray, then cook for 8 minutes. Shake once.

5. serve.

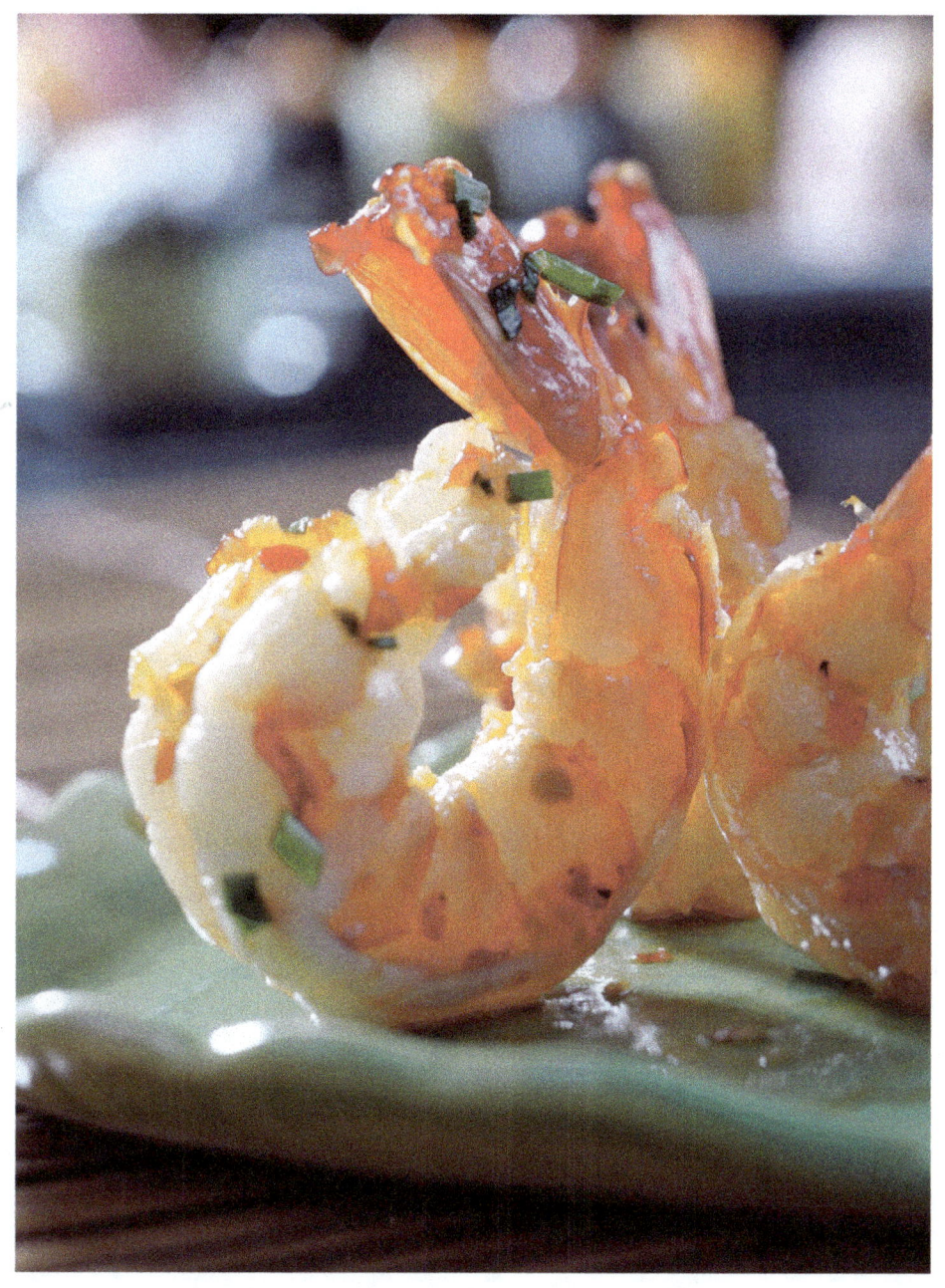

Tuna Steak

Servings: 2

- 2 (6-ounce) tuna steaks
- 1 tablespoon coconut oil, melted
- ½ teaspoon garlic powder
- **2** teaspoons white sesame seeds
- 2 teaspoons black sesame seeds

Directions:

1. Brush each tuna steak with coconut oil and sprinkle with garlic powder.
2. In a bowl, mix sesame seeds and press each tuna steak into them. Coat well.
3. Place tuna steaks into the air fryer basket.
4. Cook at 400f for 8 minutes.
5. Flip steaks halfway through the Cooking time.
6. Serve.

Trout With Butter Sauce

Servings: 2

- 2 trout fillets, boneless
- Salt and black pepper, to taste
- ½ teaspoons lemon zest, grated
- 1 ½ tablespoons chives, chopped
- 3 tablespoons butter
- 1 tablespoon olive oil
- 1 teaspoon lemon juice

Directions:

1. Season trout with salt and pepper. Drizzle with oil and rub well.
2. Cook in the air fryer at 360f for 10 minutes. Flip once.
3. Meanwhile, heat a pan with the butter over medium heat. Add lemon juice, zest, chives, salt, and pepper. Whisk well and cook for 2 minutes, then remove from heat.

4.Divide fish fillets on plates. Drizzle with butter sauce and serve.

Crab Legs In Lemon Butter

Servings: 2

- 2tablespoons salted butter, melted and divided
- 1 ½ pounds crab legs
- ¼ teaspoon garlic powder
- Juice of ½ lemon

Directions:
Drizzle 1 tablespoon butter over crab legs. Place crab legs into the air fryer basket.

Cook at 400f for 15 minutes. Flip the crab legs halfway through thecooking time.

Mix garlic powder, lemon juice, and remaining butter in a bowl.

Open crab legs and remove meat.

Dip in lemon butter and serve.

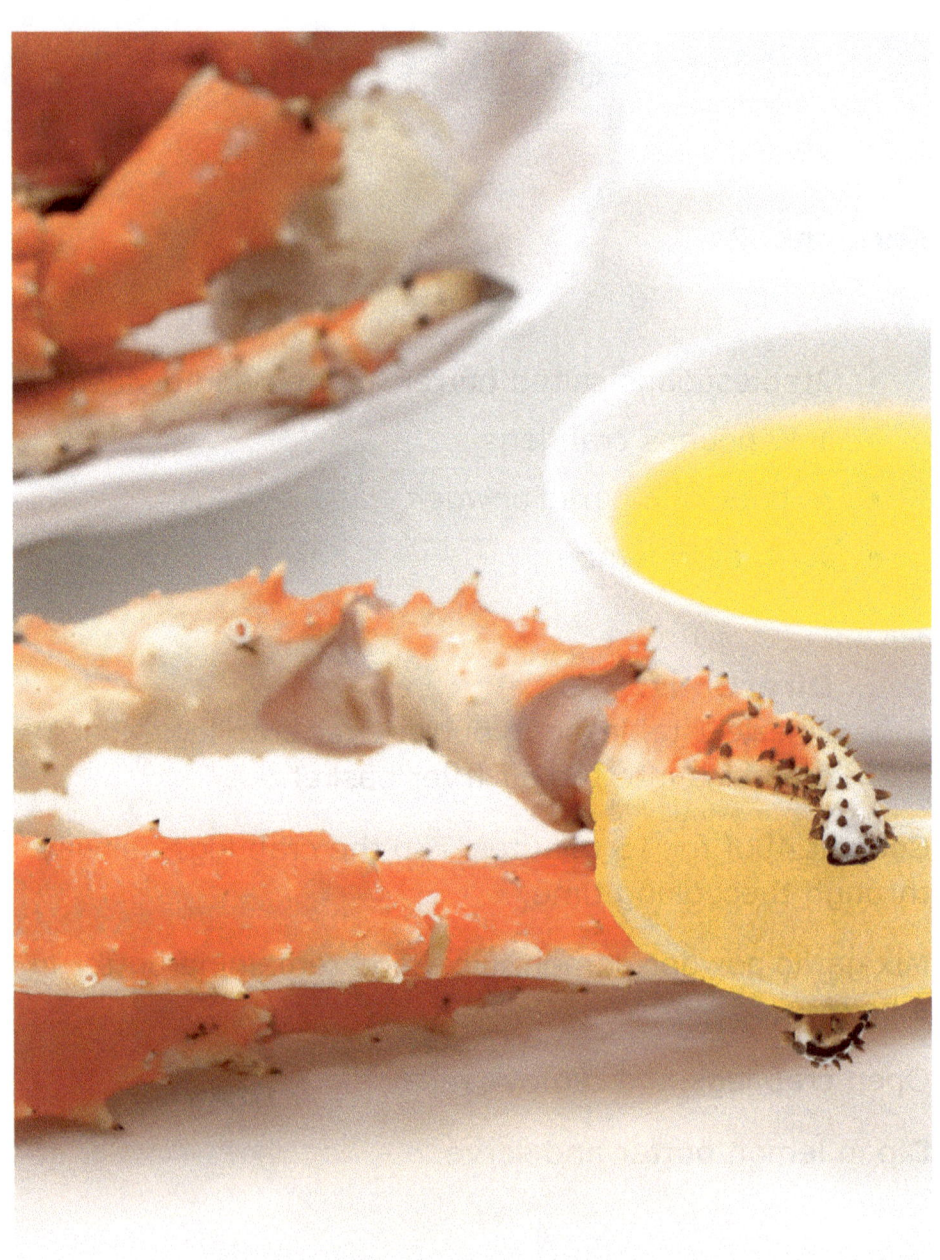

www.ingramcontent.com/pod-product-compliance
Lightning Source LLC
Chambersburg PA
CBHW070732030426
42336CB00013B/1946